When You're Hungry,
You Gotta Eat

When You're Hungry, You Gotta Eat

You Gotta Eat

The No Diet Approach to Lose Weight
and Maximize your Workout

NATHALIE PLAMONDON-THOMAS

iUniverse, Inc.
Bloomington

When You're Hungry, You Gotta Eat
The No Diet Approach to Lose Weight and Maximize your Workout

www.dnalifecoaching.com
www.dnacoachdevie.com

iUniverse books may be ordered through booksellers or by contacting:
iUniverse
1663 Liberty Drive
Bloomington, IN 47403
www.iuniverse.com
1-800-Authors (1-800-288-4677)

ISBN: 978-1-4620-5224-0 (sc)
ISBN: 978-1-4620-5225-7 (ebk)

Printed in the United States of America

iUniverse rev. date: 09/24/2011

Contents

Introduction

This book is about nutrition. I am not a dietician, doctor, or nutritionist. Remember it's me speaking, and I don't know everything. But I am curious, passionate about food, and always want to learn more.

I love food! I think about food all the time. I love cooking and I make everything from scratch.

In this book, I will try to explain to you in layman's terms how your brain processes information about hunger and satiety and how you can use that knowledge to finally achieve and maintain your optimal weight.

This book was created to help you open your mind to find your own answers to your questions. It is also designed to remind you of what you do know and motivate you to do what you know is right.

Someone told me the following one day: knowing and not doing is like not knowing at all.

1

Quiz on Myths about
Diet and Exercising

**"When hearing something often enough,
most people consider it to be the *truth*."**

Let's see if this theory has affected our knowledge of health and nutrition.

The quiz in this chapter is designed to open up the subjects that will be covered in this book.

Some answers can be true or false or both. Feel free to check both boxes. I am trying to use this quiz to remind you of the fact that there are so many studies, theories, facts, and myths about diet and exercising. We hear them over and over. So these statements serve as an introduction to what will be discussed in the rest of the book.

Take the quiz now. Let's see how you do.

Go ahead, fill in this quiz, and check your answers on the following pages.

#	Statement	TRUE	FALSE
1	It's okay to work out on an empty stomach if it's in the morning.		
2	Tea and coffee are counted in the amount of water I have to consume each day.		
3	If I have never exercised before and I want to lose weight, I should start exercising *and* cut calories from my diet.		
4	Granola bars and fruit bars are better than sports drinks during exercising.		
5	Extra-lean ground beef has less fat than ground turkey.		
6	The size of a deck of cards = 1 portion of meat.		
7	Carbohydrate turns into energy, protein turns into muscles, fat turns into fat.		
8	The best way to resist temptation is with willpower.		
9	Cravings are directed by taste buds.		
10	Your body burns most of its calories through activity.		

11	As long as food is low fat, it's not going to make you fat.		
12	Eating nuts every day will help you lose weight.		
13	Sucralose/glucose/aspartame/corn syrup/Splenda trick your mind so you stay hungry longer.		
14	Weight training is better than cardiovascular training in order to lose weight.		
15	Multi-grain bread is better than whole-grain bread because of the variety of the grains.		
16	A *light* olive oil is better than regular olive oil.		
17	The fewer ingredients on a package the better.		
18	It's okay to eat between meals.		
19	A snack that contains fewer than 100 calories is good for you.		
20	All types of cholesterol are bad.		

Answers

1. It's okay to work out on an empty stomach if it's in the morning.

FALSE

It's never okay to work out on an empty stomach. Your body needs energy in order to be able to produce the results that you want when you exercise. I am going to discuss in this book what to eat before, during, and after your workout. You will learn how you should feed yourself at least two hours before a cardiovascular exercise and one hour before strength training. But what if your workout is at 6:00 a.m.? It's not practical to get up at 4:00 a.m. just to eat. What should you do in that case? Drink a lot of water or maybe a sports drink/shake before the class. Ideally feed yourself with liquid food, rather than solid. You will see the best options later.

2. Tea and coffee are counted in the amount of water I have to consume each day.

TRUE but . . .

Here is my take on the issue of whether or not coffee, tea, and soft drinks count as water intake. Coffee, tea, and soft drinks should not count as water intake because all of these drinks contain caffeine, which is a natural diuretic. Diuretics increase the dehydration process. However, the research says that yes, as far as hydration, all liquid beverages are included in the eight to ten cups of water we need to drink daily. With that point of view, caffeine drinks, juices, soft drinks, and other drinks are also included. Soda pop is loaded with sugar, diet sodas are even worse, full of some terrible fake substances such as formaldehyde (which is used in hospitals to disinfect instruments). Caffeine drinks are not ideal. They are made with water, yes, but remember that caffeine is a diuretic, which means that it takes away one of the eight to ten cups of water a day you should drink. So if you have a coffee or tea, you need to add another cup of water to your daily intake. You need to decide what is best for you, but remember that caffeine can dehydrate you. Also be careful of soft drinks and juice, because you can accidentally take your daily intake of calories in drinks. Don't drink your calories; eat them!

3. If I have never exercised before and I want to lose weight, I should start exercising and cut calories from my diet.

FALSE

Surprise! I tricked you here. We all know that nutrition and exercise are the two components of weight loss. But the trick in this question is the *"I never exercised before"* portion. If you've never exercised before, and say your caloric intake is 2,000 calories daily, then you do a workout that burns 500 calories, *and* you cut 500 calories from your diet, that only leaves you with 1,000 calories to fuel your entire day! It's not enough. You'll be tired, and you won't have enough calories to really perform well during your workout. You will hate it and give up very quickly. That is why we see so many super-motivated people start exercising *and* cut calories at the same time, and then, a few weeks later, they give up because they are exhausted and their workouts are not giving them any results. Because we exercise, we need to make sure we have proper nutrition at the same time. Most people don't eat *enough* or don't eat *enough real food* to be able to work out efficiently. But that's another subject. The other lesson we can take from this quiz question is that by doing one thing at a time, turning it into a habit, then attacking another thing, turning it into a habit, then something else, and so on is the key for success. Some people go full on! They start exercising *and* cut calories from their diet *and* quit smoking *and* move *and* divorce *and* change jobs *and* . . . burn out! One step at a time, guys.

4. Granola bars and fruit bars are better than sports drinks during exercising.

FALSE

During a workout, you shouldn't chew. Solid food is not really recommended while exercising. Drinks can get into your system better *during* a workout. But what kinds of drinks? What about those sugar-loaded sports drinks? Are they good for you? The intention behind them is to give you the electrolytes and minerals (salt) you are losing during your workout.

I use coconut water, which contains natural electrolytes. Again, be careful, not all the brands of coconut water are the real deal. Read your labels. Some of them are also loaded with sugar.

5. Extra-lean ground beef has less fat than ground turkey.

TRUE

This is because we don't know which part of the meat was ground. A long time ago, ground beef was invented. Then came the extra lean or lean ground beef, from which some fat has been removed. Now in our minds, we know that turkey and chicken are a leaner meat than beef, naturally. But when it comes to ground meat, is there such a thing as extra-lean ground chicken or extra-lean ground turkey? Do you think they use the nice chicken breasts and the best parts of the chicken or turkey and grind it? I guess what I am saying is this: don't think you eat healthy because you buy ground chicken instead of ground beef. Be skeptical of what else has been thrown in the grinder. I am really careful when it comes to meat, and I only eat lean cuts of organic meat, in moderation. If you love ground meat, then go to the butcher and specifically ask for the breast to be ground up. Then you know what's in it.

Side note: Have you watched the *Jamie Oliver Food Revolution* when he demonstrates to children how they make chicken nuggets? Really gross. Watch it here: www.youtube.com/watch?v=S9B7im8aQjo

6. The size of a deck of cards = 1 portion of meat.

TRUE

It's all about portion sizes. Be aware of what makes up one portion. I discuss portions later in this book. How many portions per day should you eat? How much is a portion? So keep reading!

7. Carbohydrate turns into energy, protein turns into muscles, fat turns into fat.

FALSE

Carbohydrate is a source of energy for the body. The amino acids in the proteins contribute to muscle building, but you still need to do the work to create muscle. If you eat protein and sit on the couch, the proteins will certainly not turn into muscle, let me tell you that! And fat doesn't turn into fat! *Good* fat can make you leaner (for example, omega 3, essential fatty acids known as EFAs and others). Saturated fat can turn into fat. Examples of saturated fats are solid fats on meats and margarine (because they're hydrogenated). I will talk about this later on.

8. The best way to resist temptation is with willpower.

FALSE

Forget about willpower! When you're hungry, your brain tells you you're hungry. Your body is designed for one thing: survival. So your body will tell you when you are hungry until you feed yourself. Even with tons of willpower, when you are hungry, you must eat real food. The most important chapter of this book (chapter 2) will explain to you how the brain processes all the information about hunger and satiety.

9. Cravings are directed by taste buds.

FALSE

Cravings are directed by the part of the brain that handles emotion and senses, for example, your sense of smell or memories. If you crave sugar, eating a chocolate cake or a nice fresh mango will satisfy your sugar craving. It is your emotions that decide that it is the chocolate cake you want and not the mango. But these two foods will not be processed the same and not be used the same by the body. More likely, the mango will be digested and used for energy, and the chocolate cake will be stored for you to get squished a little tighter in your favourite pair of jeans. If you do indulge once in a while, use the 80/20 rule. Eat well 80 percent of the time and only indulge 20 percent of the time. And during that 20 percent, slow down . . . maximize the pleasure. Enjoy each bite slowly.

10. Your body burns most of its calories through activity.

FALSE

Just the fact of *being* burns a lot of calories! Even when you're at rest, your body needs energy for all its «hidden» functions, such as breathing, circulating blood, adjusting hormone levels, and growing and repairing cells. The number of calories your body uses to carry out these basic functions is known as your basal metabolic rate (BMR)—what you might call metabolism. According to the Mayo Clinic, your basal metabolic rate accounts for about 60 to 75 percent of the calories you burn every day.

Moving, walking, and working out add to your energy needs. That means you probably need more calories than just what is required to keep you alive.

11. As long as food is low fat, it's not going to make you fat.

FALSE

What else can make you fat? Sugar! Processed food—anything that has been refined or modified. Most packaged foods claiming to be "low-fat" are full of these sugary and refined/modified ingredients. People also tend to overeat so called low-fat foods and thus get those extra calories, which could cause weight gain.

12. Eating nuts every day will help you lose weight.	**TRUE** If you are gaining weight because your portions are too big, eating nuts will help you lose weight. Here's how. There is good fat in a nut, which sends a signal to your brain that tells you you're full. It takes about twenty minutes for the signal to make it to your brain. So eat a few nuts about twenty minutes before your meal; it will send a signal to your brain that you're full by the time you start eating. You'll keep your portions smaller. How much is a few nuts? A handful. Whatever doesn't fit in your hand is too many.
13. Sucralose / glucose / aspartame / corn syrup / Splenda trick your mind so you stay hungry longer.	**TRUE** Later in this book, I will explain the functions of grehlin and leptin, the two main hormones that control hunger and appetite. Drs. Oz and Roizen explain in their book <u>*YOU: The Owner's Manual*</u> how the sugar substitutes inhibit leptin secretion, so you never get the message that you are full. These substances break the communication between your stomach and your brain and trick your mind. You stay hungry longer when you use these types of sweeteners. Also, your body doesn't process these properly anyway because your body can't recognize them.

14. Weight training is better than cardiovascular training in order to lose weight.

TRUE or FALSE

But let's understand what each type of activity does. This is a war that has existed between the cardiovascular world and the strength training world for a number of years. We all know that we need both cardiovascular training and strength training. Let's say your body has accumulated some fat, and you want to lose it. This fat will not melt away because you pump your heart. The reason why people lose weight from cardio is because, more likely, they are working their muscles at the same time. Fat doesn't melt on its own. The strongest things in your body that can actually get rid of the fat are your muscles. When they contract, the muscles squeeze the fat away. Therefore, weight training involving good contraction will make you lose weight better and faster than cardio.

Now that being said, you do need a strong heart to work these muscles. Pumping your heart will also help improve your metabolism and make your heart stronger, which is awesome. You want your heart to be strong, as it is your primary engine. You want your metabolism to work well because a high metabolism makes you burn more calories for the same exercise. So you need to do both cardiovascular training and strength training.

15.
Multi-grain bread is better than whole-grain bread because of the variety of grains.

FALSE

Multi-grain doesn't always mean *whole* grain. You have to read the ingredients. A product needs to be made from whole grain. If it's multi-grain, it can still be all processed! So make sure you choose whole grain. This question is to make you realize the power that marketing companies have over your brain when you're buying groceries in a hurry. Don't read just the front of the package. Read all ingredients. What if the ingredient list had all *whole* grains (wheat, spelt, kamut, for example) but also contains sugar, sucralose, fructose (or any of the "ose" devils)? Is this a good bread? No! It's got *whole* flour but also other bad things. Keep switching to the next brand until you find a bread that is both whole grain and clean from other unwanted ingredients.

Side note about grains: Whole grains are complete kernels, with many health benefits. A grain contains three parts: the bran layer, the germ, and the endosperm. They all work together to boost your health. When you see the words *whole wheat* on a package, it may only contain two parts of the wheat. The words *whole grain* contains all three. So you really want to look for these exact words. In order for the Whole Grain Council of Canada to put their 100% Whole Grain Stamp on a product, all ingredients must be whole grain; no other ingredients are allowed; and the minimum whole-grain content is 16 grams. For the United States, the Whole Grain Council advise manufacturers to use the words "whole grain" in the name of a product only if the product contains more whole grain than refined grain (i.e., 51% or more of the grain is whole grain). They allow the use of the Whole Grain Stamp on products containing 8g or more of whole grain ingredients per serving—even if the product may contain more refined grain.

16. A light olive oil is better than regular olive oil.

FALSE

An oil is an oil. It will always be 9 calories per gram of fat. In fact, no oil is light. Again, the marketing companies are trying to trick your mind. When people see *light*, they think it is better for you. As we all cook with oil now, it is important to know how oils are manufactured. The same way you have switched your white refined flour to whole flour, the same way you have switched your white refined sugar to raw cane sugar, white salt to sea salt, now it's time to switch your refined oil to an unrefined, virgin oil.

There are different manufacturing processes. You want your oil to have been transformed as little as possible. A virgin, first-cold-pressed oil has been pressed at cold temperatures, slowly, to maintain all the good properties and vitamins in the oil.

Some other oils are processed really fast (creating heat in the high-speed process), which affects the properties of the oil. Manufacturers also add solvents to make the seed sweat more and to extract more oil from it. They press the seed over and over until there is nothing left in the seed. Then they need to remove that solvent. The process used to remove that solvent is called the refining process. They remove the solvent, of course, but they also remove good things such as essential fatty acids (EFAs) and vitamins (if they are not already dead because of the heat applied) that may have survived in the oil.

Once refined, the clear, drab oily substance is then given some artificial color and taste (otherwise you would not believe that it is actually sunflower oil or canola oil). It is at that stage that the word *light* comes in. So a little bit of flavour added becomes a *light* olive oil. It does not mean it's lower in fat. It means it tastes less. A virgin oil is an oil that has not been refined, and still has all its good properties.

What about *extra virgin*? Is it more virgin than just a *virgin* oil? No. The word *extra* refers to many taste characteristics that describe the quality of the fruit that is pressed. Mainly the olive. One of these elements is the amount of acidity in the olive. If the acidity is below 0.8, then an olive can enter in the line to become extra virgin olive oil. But it only refers to olives. Some marketing companies have started to put the word *extra* on many different types of oils (such as canola, sunflower, and coconut). They are just trying to trick you as you have heard the words *extra virgin* and they think that you will think their oil is better because of that word. Now you know, don't get fooled again. The words *extra* and *virgin* are two different things. A *virgin* oil is unrefined and an *extra virgin* oil refers to olive oil only, and it's mainly a measure of acidity and taste. One more thing about EFAs. They are fragile. They are affected by air, time, and heat. So you need to look for a dark glass bottle that protects the oil. It also needs to have an expiration date because the product is alive. You want to know when it will die. Would you buy milk if it had no expiration date on it? If you buy an oil with no expiration date, chances are it is already dead—and contains no good properties for you. If it's a clear plastic bottle, consider this another red flag.

For more information about healthy oils, you can contact the Leader in first-cold-pressed oils in North America: La Maison Orphee at www.maisonorphee.com.

17. The fewer ingredients on a package the better.

TRUE

Look at the ingredients list and choose the products with the fewest ingredients. For example, on a peanut butter jar, if there is a long list of ingredients, don't buy it. The only ingredient that should be on the list is peanuts. I will talk more about label reading.

18. It's okay to eat between meals.	**TRUE** Yes, in fact, that is what I propose. When you are hungry, you need to eat real food. Eat often for stable energy without sugar peaks throughout the day. You want to avoid the up-and-down energy roller-coaster. A steady flow line of energy is much more enjoyable. You will feel great all day, be less irritable, and have more concentration and focus. Use your computer and set up some reminder pop-ups in your calendar to remind yourself to drink water and to snack: *10:00 a.m. and 3:00 p.m.: Meeting with Mrs. Snack and Mr. Water.*
19. A snack that contains fewer than 100 calories is good for you.	**FALSE** You might choose a snack full of processed fat and sugar and not real food. It's not just calories to look at. Be really skeptical. Better to go with 150 calories of a real food snack than 100 calories of fake stuff.
20. All types of cholesterol are bad.	**FALSE** We have two types of cholesterol: HDL and LDL. To remember which one is which, here is my trick: H=Healthy, L=Lousy. Here is a way to understand cholesterol's role in your body as explained by Drs. Oz and Roizen in their book *YOU: The Owner's Manual.*

You have a long highway of tubes, veins, and arteries making up your circulation system. High blood pressure, high blood sugar, the effects of cigarettes, and other factors can nick the smooth inner layer of your arteries. So the LDL cholesterol starts to fill these holes. It's like putty that you put on drywall when there is a hole that needs to be filled. The LDL putty is also trying to regularize the shape of the arteries when there are some fat deposits (like the fat present in most processed foods, on the side of a steak, and in butter and shortening).

So if there is a little lump of fat sitting in your artery, the LDL adds more putty trying to create an even surface again. But this results in making the arteries smaller, clogging them. The HDL is like a spatula that you use on your putty job. The HDL comes along and "fixes" the problem LDL starts. So where do you get the HDL? That's the EFAs that I was talking about earlier.

How did you do on the quiz? These statements serve as an introduction to what will be discussed in the rest of the book. Your score doesn't really matter. The exercise was only designed to open up your mind to what is coming next.

Let's start with the hot topic: How your body works.

2

How Your Body Works

This section is the most important part of this book. When you understand how your body works, you will definitely have a much easier time making healthy choices. It just sounds good.

So let's begin. Willpower versus hormones. We accuse willpower of sabotaging our dieting efforts because it's an excuse for making bad choices. We said in Question 8 of the quiz that willpower does not help overcome hunger. That's because hunger is a biological function. Your brain will slow you down when you are hungry. A workout on an empty stomach feels hard because your brain is telling you to slow down and re-fuel. The hunger feeling is a very powerful survival instinct.

> **Cheat sheet:**
>
> Hypothalamus = satiety center
>
> Ghrelin stimulates NPY, which slows down your metabolism and increases your appetite.
>
> Leptin stimulates CART, which increases your metabolism and slows down your appetite.
>
> But in order to do this, you need good and real food to get these signals working.

In your brain is an area in the hypothalamus called the satiety center. That's the area where your brain processes the hunger information. There are two different types of players in this area. The eating chemicals driven by NPY (a protein called neuropeptide Y) and the satiety chemicals led by CART (cocaine-amphetamine-regulatory transcript). NPY decreases metabolism and increases appetite. CART stimulates the surrounding hypothalamus to increase metabolism, reduce appetite, and increase insulin to deliver energy to muscle cells rather than be stored as fat.

When you are hungry, NPY will slow you down. It will not let you use your energy because it is afraid you will run out of fuel. So it slows your metabolism down. You have an empty stomach, you are starting your workout and somehow you don't feel like it's going to be a good workout. You just can't feel the energy, and you feel weaker than normal. You hear messages in your mind like *I don't know what is going on, I'm doing the same workout as usual, but today is so much harder.* You then start wanting to eat. Your brain is telling you to slow down because it's in need of energy. The light of your gas gauge is on—you need fuel. NPY increases your appetite.

The CART is the reverse. When you have enough food in your stomach, these brain chemicals send the brain a signal to increase your metabolism. The body is ordered to increase the level of energy. And your brain receives a signal that now the stomach is full of energy, so it tells the body to go ahead, spend some energy, I'm good to go, I have a full tank! Then you can start running and working out with energy, or you can go back to work after a healthy lunch and start to concentrate again, see things clearly, and move with vigor. CART decreases your appetite. You need some good food in order for your brain to receive the signal that it's okay to start moving again.

Who is giving these signals to the brain?

The grehlin and the leptin. They are both stress hormones, and they work with the NPY and the CART.

The grehlin works hand in hand with the NPY. When you have used up your fuel, the grehlin will transmit the signal to the NPY area of the brain. (I call it the gremlin to remind myself which one is which.) The grehlin is the little voice that tells the brain: *I'm hungry.* Have you ever heard that voice? Of course you have. Because as a human, the very first instinct is always to survive. So when you are hungry, you will hear that grehlin tell you every thirty minutes, then every twenty minutes, then every fifteen, ten . . . and then soon, if you still don't feed yourself, eating will be the one sole thing in your mind.

The leptin is the satisfactory hormone. It will stimulate the CART. It will get information from your stomach and notice if it is being fueled. When it notices real food in the stomach, it will give the message to the CART area of the brain to say that it's okay to move and spend energy again.

You can read more about the anatomy of appetite in the book by Drs. Oz and Roizen called *YOU: On a Diet.*

In Layman's Terms

That was the scientific part of the book . . . done! Now, let's see if I can explain that to you again in my own words. Not that my vocabulary is so great.

> **You can't trick your body!**
>
> It will notice if you eat real food versus junk. Processed foods are not recognized by your body as a real food, so your body stores it! So you're still hungry and take in more calories.

This mechanism only works with real food. Your body is smart. Your brain is smart. Go figure. I hope so because if the brain is not smart, then what is? Your body notices what you eat. Surprise! You can't just put a chocolate bar in your mouth and hope that your body will not notice. It will.

Let's say, for example, it's lunch time. You had breakfast before work, you may even have had a snack, an apple, a rice cake, or something similar around 10:00 a.m. and now you're ready for lunch. Yet you have not brought your lunch with you. So you go to your favorite coffee shop and get a ham and cheese sandwich. It tastes great, and you feel full.

But what does your body say? Your gremlin (grehlin) is yelling, asking for food. It sees this sandwich coming in. So it says *great*! I love ham and cheese sandwiches. What's this? Bread. Cool! Fiber and carbs are coming. But wait a minute. Your body doesn't recognize the refined and processed white bread, so it decides to just put it aside for now and stores it—on your butt, your thighs, your stomach, anywhere it can. The grehlin keeps asking for more food.

But what about the ham? That's protein, right? But, it's processed ham, and again your body doesn't recognize it. It decides to store that too. Next we have some cheese. Great! Dairy and protein together! But it's processed cheese, and your body doesn't know what it is. What does it do with it? Stores it! Same with the mayo.

So the grehlin keeps asking for more and more food and will not shut up until you actually feed it. At the end of your lunch, all you've really eaten is a slice of tomato and a piece of lettuce! Vegetables. But with that you're only good for a few minutes. It's no wonder you are hungry again in an hour. You haven't actually been fed properly.

So what do you do at the end of the meal with that gremlin still yelling for food in your brain? You go get an oatmeal-raisin cookie. A bit of oat will help and a few raisins are good, but all the refined sugar will be stored with the rest of the junk. So, really, lots of garbage just added to the pile of unwanted inches covering your body. It's just stuffing yourself with "stuff" that is not real.

One more important detail

Your body learns from your cravings and adapts to how long you normally take to feed it.

Be organized and have a plan about how many calories you want to allow yourself for a healthy and balanced diet. Spread them throughout the day. Decide when you want to be hungry and stick to the plan. Your body will adapt.

It is really amazing how quickly you can change a bad habit. When you get the first signal, ask yourself if you are really hungry. Or is this a bad habit that you used to give in to at the first sign of hunger?

Have a glass of water. You might just be thirsty. If hunger persists, then it means it is the real grehlin signal. Then it's time for your planned snack.

Make sure you eat a real food snack!

Now keep your attention on the next lines because we are not done here. Some of you are thinking right now that it's okay to store some garbage stuff when you work out a lot. You think that the stuff accumulated on your bum at lunch time will get out at 6:00 p.m. when you hit the gym.

I'm sorry to have to be the one telling you the hard truth. With no proper fuel, when you do your workout, you crash. Your workout does not fix the problems you ate.

As an example, when you are hungry yourself, do you open the refrigerator door or the garbage can to look for food? You want fresh, good energy, right? When your body needs fuel, it looks for good fuel. So it won't take the fat/garbage that it did not want in the first place. It stored it once. It will not run to the garbage at the first sign of hunger. If you are not eating it, you are stealing it from your body. If the glycogen store is empty, your body will look for protein for fuel. It might take some energy from your muscles and bones, and then your workout makes you actually weaker than you were before. It will shrink your muscles, making you lose muscle mass, not fat. The garbage will still be there, but the muscles will be shrinking, changing your body composition.

So how do you get rid of your garbage? You need to contract your muscles so they get rid of the accumulated fat. Therefore, it is really important that you feed yourself before your workout. Real food. You have to have the energy to squeeze properly.

A Big Dinner But Not Fed

I went out for dinner with my husband to one of our favorite Italian restaurants. We like pasta, and that is one of the reasons why I make my own pasta because I can control what kind of flour I use. Restaurants usually use white refined flour, unfortunately. So at that Italian restaurant they did. The meal tasted fantastic! We started with the bread dipped in extra virgin olive oil and balsamic vinegar. Yum! Then we had some pasta for our meal. And as a treat, we shared a chocolate cake for dessert.*

> ***Remember**
>
> 80/20 rule applies here:
>
> If 80 percent of the time you are good, then you can treat yourself the other 20 percent of the time.
>
> The more you follow this rule, the more healthy treats you will find and the more your taste will change for better food. So you won't crave the bad stuff as often and the percentage will more likely change to 90/10 or 95/5 without effort, until your idea of a treat becomes a medjool date or a fresh mango.

We walked back home from the Italian restaurant absolutely stuffed. But yet, when we got home, I made myself a peanut butter toast before bed. My husband looked at me and said, "Are you crazy? We just ate a huge meal!"

But the problem is that I had not been properly fed. The bread was white bread, the pasta was white pasta, and we all know there is nothing healthy in chocolate cake. There was nothing I had in my meal that actually fed my body. It tasted great, and I loved it, but I had to teach a fitness class in the morning, and I knew I couldn't do it if I didn't feed my body. You have to make up for your mistakes, and that doesn't mean starving yourself because starving doesn't help. It means getting back on track to fueling your body properly. So you can work out properly and get rid of the "improper stuff."

Fresh pasta

One of the reasons why I make my own pasta (other than the fact that fresh homemade pasta is absolutely to die for) is that I can control the type of flour that I use and what I put in it.

A real whole flour pasta really feeds you well, and you actually don't need that much. A portion the size of your fist should do it.

You should have seen my husband's face the very first time I made homemade pasta. He was excited, having participated in the making of it, and he was looking forward to a big bowl of homemade pasta. He was so sorry when he saw the size of plate I brought him. "That's it?" he said with a pitiful face, "That's all I'm getting?" Well guess what? Even if it was delicious, a real homemade pasta with whole flour fills you up much quicker than the regular white flour processed pasta. So not only is the melt-in-your-mouth taste much better, you also eat less because real food actually feeds you.

3

Why Eat? Why Exercise?

Why should we eat food? We need food to give us energy. Food provides us with three major things: carbohydrates, proteins, and lipids, which are the main building blocks of nutrition. Food also gives us vitamins and minerals (more like extra protection, like your insurance policy).

Vitamins and minerals are even more important for people who exercise. When we exercise, we tend to be hard on our bodies, creating a by-product of exercise

What are the 3 things that we need to be healthy?

- Healthy eating
- Healthy exercising
- Healthy thinking

This book mainly talks about eating and exercising. For the healthy thinking part, see Nathalie's new Seminar called Think Yourself Thin at DNA Life Coaching, http://www.dnalifecoaching.com/category/events/.

called lactic acid. Now, I want to make sure that I am clear here. I am not saying that exercising isn't good for you. It is one of the three major things we actually need in life in order to be healthy. But because we exercise, and even though we get all the benefits from exercise that we will talk about below, we also are more in need of vitamins and minerals. They provide antioxidants and help to protect us because we do a lot to our bodies.

About ten years ago, I discovered a comprehensive self-help book that changed the way I see food and supplements: *Prescription for Nutritional Healing* by James F. Balch, MD, and Phyllis A. Balch, CNC. Their book taught me that there is always a natural solution to any health problem we might face. I have bought many new editions of this book over the years, and I constantly refer to it for whatever is going on. It's easy to search for subjects because they are classified in alphabetical order. For example, if I have a headache, I go to the letter H index to see what I can eat that will help. If I have a bruise, I will look in the letter B section to see how I can fix or avoid it next time.

Why should we train? We need to train for cardiovascular health and muscular strength. We need a strong heart that can pump life in our bodies, and we need strong muscles that will take us everywhere we want to go and do anything we want to do.

We also need to train because of the change in lifestyle that our society is going through. We've taken activity out of daily living. For example, as a population, we no longer take stairs, we take elevators. We don't manually file, squatting to open the heavy drawers, we computer file instead with our mouse. We don't cut our vegetables, we buy them all pre-cut for us. We don't roll the windows down in our cars, we just press a button. We don't open doors anymore, they are all automated. We don't burn as many calories in daily activities as our ancestors did years ago.

The following chart shows all the calories we *don't* burn during our daily activities and how we can gain 12 pounds a year:

The Calories We Don't Burn Anymore

You can see, in the following table, the results of a research on difference in caloric expenditure conducted in 1993, on clerical workers, weighing in average 150 lb. They compared with the same task done in 1953.

At Work

Now	Then	Result: (fewer calories burned)
Elevator	Stairs	3,900 cal/year
Computer filing	Manual filing	2,400 cal/year
Keyboard	Manual typing	9,600 cal/year
		15,900 cal/year = 4.5 lb / year

Transportation

Now	Then	Result: (fewer calories burned)
Driving	Walking	3,780 cal/year
Automatic transmission	Manual transmission	2,700 cal/year
Power windows, brakes, auto wash	Manual	900 cal/year
		7,380 cal/year = 2.1 lb / year

At Home

Now	Then	Result: (fewer calories burned)
Food processor, mixer, pre-cut vegetables, pre-washed	Hand chopping / mashing/ washing / can opening	3,600 cal/year
Dishwasher	Hand washing	6,205 cal/year
Remote control	TV, stereo, garage door	4,052 cal/year
Power mower / snow blower	Hand mower / shovel	4,320 cal/year
		18,177 cal/year = 5.2 lb / year

Total calories we don't burn anymore

Work	15,900 cal/year 4.5 lb / year
Transportation	7,380 cal/year 2.1 lb / year
Home	18,177 cal/year 5.2 lb / year
= 800 cal/week	**41,457 cal/year = 11,8 lb / year!**

So we gain 12 pounds per year just because we live in today's world! And that study was done almost 20 years ago. Can you image what it would be nowadays?

4

Let's Talk About Weight Management

First, there is no ideal weight. The number on the scale does not matter. We worry too much about this number. A muscle is much heavier than fat. So when you lose fat, your scale number might actually increase!

A lot of people decide they want to lose weight because of the number on the scale. That's not the right way to approach it. You should want to lose weight because it would be dangerous for you not to. The only number that matters is your waist measurement. Accumulating weight around your waist, in your stomach, is really the key here. See the Body Types Note.

Body types

There are two different body types: apple and pear. Of the two, which is healthier?

It's less dangerous to have a big butt with the pear shape. But gaining weight in the stomach area is dangerous. Fat accumulates around your heart, liver, organs, and digestive system. This is the apple shape.

The fat that accumulates there starts to put pressure on your organs.

It's dangerous for your health to be apple-shaped, and you should want to lose weight for your health.

How many calories do I need each day?

The following exercise will give you an idea of a correct number of calories you should eat to maintain your current weight or to lose a few pounds. For precise meal planning, there are more detailed measures and calculations needed. This will simply help you to understand where you need to cut calories if you are looking to lose weight. This exercise is interesting as it helps you realize how many calories you should actually put in your mouth. If you have an idea of how many calories you should eat in a day, it makes you think a little longer before you swallow that 1,100-calorie fruit smoothie.

Instructions for filling out the sheet:

Fill out the following worksheet. Take your actual weight, multiply by 10. This gives you the ideal daily caloric intake to sustain your weight and self.

BMR (Basic Metabolic Rate) can be hard to guess. If you're really active, you might be a 0.6. Otherwise you might be a 0.4 if you exercise regularly but not super intensely. If you don't work out, your rate might be 0.2.

Multiply the BMR by your ideal daily caloric intake to get the number of extra calories you need to consume to sustain yourself.

Then you get your ideal daily caloric intake that takes into consideration your activity level.

The purpose is not to start counting and calculating everything you eat. This exercise gives you an idea of how and where to get your calories, so you can see where you need to increase or decrease.

I've put in an example in parentheses for you to see. Fill in your own information.

Current Weight	(135)	×	10	(1350)	Ideal Daily Caloric Intake
BMR (Basic Metabolic Rate)	0.4	×	(1350)	(540)	Average activity factor 40%
OR BMR (Basal Metabolic Rate)	0.6	×	(1350)	(810)	Average activity factor 60%
Ideal Daily Caloric Intake	(1350)	+	(810)	(If BMR = 0.4 1890 calories)	(If BMR = 0.6 2160 calories)

What Is the Deficit Required to Lose Weight?

How many calories make up one pound of weight? That's 3,500 calories! To lose weight healthily and safely, you should lose no more than one pound per week. What does that look like in terms of daily caloric intake? Here's another worksheet to help you.

Note: Only complete this sheet for the first 10 pounds you want to lose. Do not do more than 10 pounds at a time, because your weight and caloric intake will change as you lose weight. Recalculate after you have lost your first 10 pounds, and add in the next 10 pounds. Do only 10 pounds at a time.

Once you know how many calories you need to eat, you can try to make your own program or see a nutritionist or a nutrition and wellness specialist who is knowledgeable in this area. You can immerse yourself in the

Remember

This is just a guide. Every person is different.

I was working with a young professional lacrosse player in Toronto who was only 5 feet 1 inch tall and wanted to lose 5 pounds. She was 90 pounds. She had been 85 pounds most of her life and had splurged on her mom's baking over the holiday season and could not seem to get these 5 pounds off.

Her daily caloric intake was around 1400. So if we take off 500, that means she only has 900 calories per day!

Nobody can survive on that, so we modified the program, and the athlete lost half a pound per week, instead of one pound.

You must make adjustments for your own body.

calorie world if you would like, but be careful to make sure you don't look just at caloric intake. You *must* eat real food and a variety of it. A good example is burgers and fries that can be the same number of calories as a salad with avocados and lean protein and spinach. Some people will put the burger in their planner thinking that it's the same number of calories. Or put a diet soft drink instead of fresh juice on their planner because it has zero calories. Be really careful.

Again, my example is in parentheses for you to see. Fill in your own information.

Pounds to lose	(10)	×	3500	(35000)	Calories deficit total
1 pound / week	1	×	3500	3500	Calories deficit per week
Daily calories deficit	3500	/	7	500	Daily calories
Low activity day	(1890) (from table above)	-	500	(1390)	1200 minimum!
High activity day	(2160) (from table above)	-	500	(1660)	

Note the 1200 minimum. Why? Because you still need your energy! You should not go below 1200 calories per day.

5

What the "Bleep" Can You Eat?

Now that you know the average number of calories that you should be eating daily, you need to know how to get these calories. The very first rule is eat real food! And when you're not hungry anymore, stop eating. Eat a variety of food. And nothing processed.

If you focus on what you *can* eat, and you eat *real* food, you will not be hungry. It will be plenty of food. So what should be on your list?

A side note about fiber

Fiber is part of your carbs, but it doesn't give you energy to exercise. Fiber is not transformed into energy.

It's kind of a filter. Every other food you eat during the day gets filtered through the fiber. How cool is that?

So ideally we don't eat fiber late at night. Eat it in the morning to start the filter and make you feel fuller longer.

- Protein: 0.38 × your weight or about 50 to 100 g per day
- Carbohydrates (complex versus simple): 40 percent of your diet
- Fiber (25 g for women, 38 g for men)
- Limit simple sugar intake to 4 g per meal
- Lipids (fats): 20-35 percent of your diet
- Limit saturated fat intake to 4 g per meal

- Vitamins and minerals
  - o Including calcium 1000-1200 mg / day
  - o Including vitamin D 600 IU / day to assimilate the calcium
  - o You can choose to eat your vitamins through your food or to take supplements. But remember that taking vitamins as a supplement does not compensate for a bad diet.
- Water

What is the deal with food combinations? Should we eat some food first? Last? Together? Mostly, it doesn't matter. It's good to have fiber in the morning as mentioned earlier, as it will be used as a filter for the rest of the food intake of the day. Also, eating protein along with carbohydrates will make the carbs last longer, so spread your protein intake to have some at every meal.

6

Portions: How Much Should You Eat?

Here are the number of portions you should eat daily:

o   Fruits and vegetables: 7 to 10 portions per day
o   Grain products: 6 to 8 portions per day
o   Dairy and substitutes: 2 to 3 portions per day
o   Meat and substitutes: 2 to 3 portions per day
o   Oils: 2 to 3 tablespoons per day
o   Water: 8 to 10 glasses per day

You should spread these throughout the day filling your plate this way:

½ with veggies
¼ with protein
¼ with starch

How much is a portion?

Pasta: your fist
Lean red meat: computer mouse
Muffin: standard light bulb
Fish: eyeglass case
Dry cereal: small white wine glass
Chocolate: package of dental floss
Rice (cooked): cupcake wrapper
Frozen yogurt: baseball
Low-fat cheese: pink eraser
Bagel: small can of tuna
Vegetable oil or mayo: a quarter
Vegetables: small scoop of ice cream
Potato: bar of soap
Fresh fruit: tennis ball
Nuts: 2 egg cups

Then use your snack to fill up the gaps with the food that you missed during your meals.

A few notes about portion sizes: One portion of cheese is a pink eraser? Yes, that's it. Savour it, spread it thinly on a thin rice cake and put salsa on it. It's a low amount. I don't even drink milk because I want to save all my dairy allowance for cheese. What's the rule with cheese? Choose a cheese that is 25 percent MF (milk fat) or less. Examples: Bocconcini, 18% MF, ricotta instead of cream cheese (it can be as low as 7%), and cottage cheese 2%.

Pasta portion is the size of your fist. That may seem small, but if it's real food (that is, made with whole wheat flour or spelt), then it will fill you up enough. Add a ton of vegetables to it, and they'll fill you up too. Consider using quinoa in pasta sauce instead of meat. It has far fewer calories and a ton more vitamins and minerals as well as protein. Its texture is similar to ground beef. I also make shepherd's pie and meat loaf with quinoa. When I use it in spaghetti sauce, I pour it over spaghetti squash (instead of pasta).

Side note about dairy

There is an interesting concept about dairy in Rory Freedman and Kim Barnouin's book *Skinny Bitch.* They say that cow milk, by design, grows a 90-pound calf into a 2,000-pound cow over the course of two years. They are also linking dairy to a host of other problems too. This book makes you re-think your dairy choices as well as the whole vegetarian and vegan idea.

The Omnivore's Dilemma by Michael Pollan is also a great book on the subject.

A rice portion is a cupcake wrapper. Start using smaller plates and start eating real brown rice. If it's real, it's filling!

Fruits and vegetables provide lots of antioxidants, which we need because we work out. Remember: a banana equals two portions of fruit. And half your plate should be vegetables.

7

Food and Training

How do you battle hunger after a workout if you're trying to lose weight? It can be difficult to lose body fat when you are trying to keep up the energy to fulfill your weekly training commitments.

Have you ever experienced *huge* after-workout hunger? You need to be prepared. Always know what will be your after-workout snack and prepare it in advance. Carry it in your gym bag. Otherwise, you will get out of the gym and won't even make it home. The hunger will attack you, and you will grab anything (good or bad) that presents itself to you.

Another thing to know about is the gym reward syndrome: You feel as if you are allowed a reward for working out. You just burned 400 calories, so you might as well get that fancy coffee with whipped cream and a shot of vanilla and that Danish right? And 800 calories later, you are up 400 calories after your workout. If you had not worked out, you wouldn't have allowed the stuff you put in your mouth after.

Be careful not to undo everything you work so hard for at the gym. That means don't overdo it in calories so you have a harder time losing weight. I often hear that from participants in my classes: *I have been coming to the gym for months. I feel that I am getting stronger but am not losing weight, nor fat.* If that sounds like you, look closely at your gym reward syndrome.

What to Eat Before Training

Avoid solid food for at least one hour before any class, or two hours before a mid—to high-impact cardio class. If you're exercising early in the morning, you may not be able to eat two hours before your workout. So drink something before the class such as a sports drink/shake. Bananas work for me in the morning before a workout. I usually make a banana shake with protein powder and water.

If you work out at 6 p.m., you should have a snack around 4 p.m. Have low glycemic index meal—the type of carbs that produces only small fluctuations in our blood glucose and insulin levels—before endurance exercise. It will improve your performance. Avoid high-fat meals because fat slows down the digestion and stomach-emptying process.

Try to stick to moderate fiber and protein, for example:

- Pasta-based meals (whole grain)
- Rolled oats such as muesli or oatmeal

> **Remember your water**
>
> Drink eight to ten glasses per day—not including the water you take at your workout. You must drink water on top of your workout to replace the water you lose in your workout.

- A skim milk or water smoothie with fruit
- Natural yogurt with fresh fruit
- A whole-grain bread sandwich with lean protein and salad filling
- Rice cakes with peanut butter or ricotta and salsa (my favorite)

What to Eat While Training

Water, water, water! Water is the best drink, certainly prior to exercise and during exercise of less than ninety minutes. If exercising more than ninety minutes, or if you tend to sweat heavily, then a sports drink is a good idea.

> **Coconut water: A great natural sports drink**
>
> Not to be confused with coconut milk. Coconut water is taken from young coconuts and is clear. The milk comes from more mature coconuts. Coconut water is a natural thirst-quencher that will help you rehydrate without all the added sugar of some sports drinks. Be aware of the imitation kinds with added sugar.

Sports drinks contain sodium, which stimulates absorption and decreases urine output. Together, these effects encourage better re-hydration than water alone. Also try gels if you're a runner, but remember to make sure they are made with good, clean ingredients. I use coconut water. Unlike the sports drinks, it is natural and clean.

What to Eat After Training

Remember two things:

- Within thirty minutes of your workout, you must have carbs. Carry something with you to make sure you replenish—a fruit or something to get those carbs in within the thirty minutes. Muscle tissue is like a sponge, with big holes, and it's wide open right after your workout. You need to fill the holes (with carbs) right after, or the next workout will feel "crunchy." It won't work as well.

- Within two hours after strength training, and sometimes after cardio, you need to eat protein. So you often have time to get home to do this.

8

Antioxidants

We need antioxidants to fight the lactic acid that the muscles produce when working out. Antioxidants combat free radicals released during exercise that can compromise your body's natural defense. Also avoid overtraining. Think of colorful foods. Some examples of great antioxidants are these:

- Squash
- Tomatoes
- Carrots
- Pomegranate
- Blueberries
- Olive oil
- Gac (a powerful fruit from Southeast Asia with more vitamin C and lycopene than oranges and carrots)

A note about diet soda

Many people consume diet soda to avoid ingesting a lot of sugar. Avoiding too much sugar is a good thing, but not when you replace it with aspartame.

Aspartame is terrible: it tricks your brain into thinking you need more food calories, so you end up overeating and gaining weight, not losing it! Your body can't recognize the aspartame, or any artificial sweeteners.

If you like soft drinks, look for carbonated water mixed with real juice (remember, real food, not artificial). Spritzers are a great alternative for sodas. Also try carbonated water with a squeeze of lemon or lime instead.

I take some vitamin supplements, for bones, for joints, for antioxidants. Even if I eat well, I also do work out a lot. So these vitamins are like my insurance policy.

9

Read Your Labels

When buying food, make sure you read your labels. Even if someone tells you that they like a particular brand of crackers or juice, don't believe them immediately. Read it for yourself. Aim for constantly increasing your knowledge.

Understanding the load of information that is shovelled to you each day is your best way of staying healthy. Even if your doctor is telling you to eat slices of fake cheese because it's a portion of dairy, don't believe it. Check for yourself. Even if the ad on TV says that the hazelnut chocolate spread contains proteins and should be given to kids, check out the remaining ingredients. Don't trust anyone. Read your labels!

Make sure to eat real food only. Check that everything listed is pronounceable and that you actually know what it is.

Added sugar is in abundance in almost all pre-packaged foods. It causes cravings and addictions to foods with no nutritional value. Stay away from the "ose" ingredients such as glucose, fructose, sucrose, dextrose, and others. Use natural sugars instead: maple syrup, honey, stevia, and agave.

When reading the package, don't just look at the number of calories or grams of fat. Look at the entire ingredient list. The shorter the ingredient list, the better. You should recognize the ingredients. If you don't, chances are that it's not real food! Eat real food. Consume food that looks the same as when it was growing.

Shop around the outside edges of the supermarket. These are the produce, dairy, and meat departments. The aisles are where the pre-packaged and processed foods are. These are often made up of ingredients that are not real food.

10

Should You Eat Organic?

You decide when it's important to buy organic. Sometimes you can't afford it or it doesn't make sense. But try to eat organic when you can.

My husband and I decided a long time ago that it did not matter what kind of car we drove, what kind of house we lived in, or what brand of clothes we wore: what matters to us is what we put in our bodies. Our health is what matters the most. What man, old and rich, and sick, would not give all his fortune for health? At home, we eat organic.

As a start, you can try to get your produce organic. Some produce is more likely to be sprayed with pesticides, so you should try to buy

The 20 fruits and veggies with the most pesticides

Some produce you should always buy organic to avoid pesticides. Ranked in order by the Environmental Working Group (EWG) with the worst at the top are peaches.

1. Peaches
2. Apples
3. Sweet bell peppers
4. Celery
5. Nectarines
6. Strawberries
7. Cherries
8. Pears
9. Grapes (imported)
10. Spinach
11. Lettuce
12. Potatoes
13. Carrots
14. Green beans
15. Hot peppers
16. Cucumbers
17. Raspberries
18. Plums
19. Grapes (domestic)
20. Oranges

them organic. If you can't afford to buy all your fruit organic, see the list in the sidebar.

Regardless, *wash* your food, even if it's organic. It has touched other things in the store, in your car, on the delivery truck, and it was touched by other people too.

The 20 fruits and veggies with the least pesticides

According to EWG, the following produce has the lowest pesticide load, ranked in order with the produce with the absolute lowest pesticides first.

1. Onion
2. Avocado
3. Sweet corn (frozen)
4. Pineapples
5. Mango
6. Asparagus
7. Sweet peas (frozen)
8. Kiwi
9. Bananas
10. Cabbage
11. Broccoli
12. Papaya
13. Blueberries
14. Cauliflower
15. Winter squash
16. Watermelon
17. Sweet potatoes
18. Tomatoes
19. Honeydew melon
20. Cantaloupe

11

Tips and Meal Ideas

Here are a few examples of easy meals I like to eat:

Breakfast

- Oatmeal (not the packaged stuff, just mix plain oats with boiling water) sweetened with a few raisins or cranberries or fresh berries
- Cereals with unsweetened soy milk:
  - Ezekiel cereals by Food for Life
  - Smart Bran with psyllium cereals by Nature's Path
  - Optimum Slim by Nature's Path
  - Silver Hills Squirrelly or Max Flax or Big 16 toast with Nuts to You peanut butter

> **My favorite salads**
>
> **Watermelon salad**
> Watermelon in cubes
> Feta cheese in cubes
> Cucumbers in cubes
> Olive oil 1 tbs
> Red wine vinegar 1 tbs
> Maple syrup 1 tbs
> Basil
> Sea salt
> Fresh ground pepper
> Serve in half watermelon as bowl
>
> **Mango salad**
> Spinach
> Fresh cilantro
> Mango
> Fish sauce ½ tsp
> Rice vinegar 2 tbs
> Sunflower oil 2 tbs
> Maple syrup 2 tbs
> Sea salt
> Fresh ground pepper

- Protein shake with banana or frozen fruit, water, flaxseed oil

Snacks

- Real Food Corn Thins rice cakes with 7% ricotta cheese and salsa
- Sun-Rype Fruit to Go Fruit bars
- Granola Bars by Kashi
- Half avocado with Raincoast tuna mixed with plain greek yogurt (instead of mayo) in the pit-hole
- Veggie sticks (always have them ready in the fridge as you most likely won't start peeling carrots or cutting cauliflower when you just want to nibble on something)
- Medjol dates
- Pecans, walnuts, almonds, pistachio (make a blend with balsamic vinegar and sea salt and add dried cranberries, dates, and other goodies)
- Protein shake/smoothie made with water

Lunch

- One of my favorite salads (see sidebar)

Couscous salad
Couscous
Pistachios
Cranberries
Raisins
Bocconcine
Cherry tomatoes
Olive oil 2 tbs
Red wine vinegar 2 tbs
Maple syrup 2 tbs
Sea salt
Fresh ground pepper

Spinach Salad
Spinach
Avocado
Hearts of palm
Tomato
Sprouts (broccoli, peas, alfalfa)
Walnut oil 2 tbs
Balsamic vinegar 2 tbs
Maple syrup 2 tbs
Sea salt
Fresh ground pepper

- Acorn squash or butternut squash soup (simply steam and puree in blender), add Belsoy dairy-free cream and fresh basil
- Pita bread sandwich with chickpeas, sprouts, spinach, avocado, tomato, plain Greek yogurt
- Grilled organic chicken breasts, cut in cubes and stored in individual portions in mini bags to add meat to any vegetarian choices (I do eat meat as well once in a while.)

Dinner

- Chickpeas (put in a slow cooker in the morning with water and onion, so they are ready for dinner) with butternut squash and yams in cubes, curry powder
- Brown rice or quinoa (pop into a rice cooker with the vegetables in the veggie steamer on top to be ready when you get back from a fitness class, and by the time you get out of the shower, the rice and the veggies are ready)
- Veggie burgers (quinoa, shredded carrots, zucchini, mushrooms, egg) with Portobello mushroom as a bun
- Lentils, lima beans, split pea stews with veggies (again, slow cooked)
- Spaghetti squash cut in half with mushrooms in the hole served with homemade quinoa spaghetti sauce (I also use quinoa to make meat loafs or sometimes I mix the quinoa with half of organic extra-lean ground beef if I have meat eaters coming over.)
- A nice piece of wild fish grilled with salad and veggies

- Homemade pizza on pita bread with ricotta cheese, chicken, shredded carrots, onion, mushrooms, Bocconcini cheese, tomatoes and peppers on top

Desserts:

- Fruit (mango is my favorite)
- Greek yogurt with fruit
- Belsoy puddings (dairy-free)
- Raspberry pie (crust made with cereals in the blender and coconut oil, tapioca starch and fresh raspberries, plain Greek yogurt on top sweetened with maple syrup)
- Having people over and want a traditional decadent dessert but you don't have time to cook? Try Pamela's Wheat-Free and Gluten-Free Chocolate Brownie Mix or Classic Vanilla Cake Mix.

Some Final Tips

- Eat often—every two to three hours (complex carbs and lean proteins) and drink water.
- Fiber and fat (essential fatty acids) are your best buddies.
- Eat at home. Keep a full fridge or use a cooler to go.
- Prepare, Prepare, Prepare!
- Use smaller plates to help control portion sizes (9-inch plates).
- *Never* skip breakfast and *never* starve.
- Exercise four to five times a week (with others).
- Set up short-term goals and tell the whole world! It will help you commit to your plan. Tell people you don't eat garbage—at work, at home, or socially.

- Take "before" pictures and measurements.
- Avoid refined, processed, and sugar-loaded foods.
- *Eat real food!* Complement with vitamins and supplements.

My Favorite Things

> ### Duff!
>
> It's important that you have someone who supports you. For me, it's my husband, Duff. For you, it may be a friend, child, or spouse. You must be on board together.

- Aluminum water bottle and bottle shaker
- Vegetable steamer / rice cooker
- Slow cooker
- Maple syrup (that is my sugar of choice)
- Rice cakes (I like the thin ones)
- Spinach
- Walnuts, almonds, nuts
- Bocconcini cheese, feta cheese, ricotta cheese
- Quinoa
- Eggs—boil them and keep them in their shells in the fridge for a handy protein (no more than five eggs per week)
- Walnut oil (first-cold-pressed traditional recipe from La Maison Orphee)
- Balsamic vinegar
- My protein shake
- Fruit To Go—mini bites by Sun-Rype
- Beans and peas
- Dates
- Avocado
- Insulated grocery bags with zipper
- A grocery list

REMEMBER:

Knowing and not doing
is like
not knowing at all.

Now you know . . . What are you going to do?

Helpful References

Balch, James F., MD, and Phyllis A. Balch, CNC, *Prescription for Nutritional Healing: A Practical A-to-Z Reference to Drug-Free Remedies Using Vitamins, Minerals, Herbs and Food Supplements* (New York: Avery, 2006).

Freedman, Rory, and Kim Barnouin, *Skinny Bitch: A No-Nonsense, Tough-Love Guide for Savvy Girls Who Want to Stop Eating Crap and Start Looking Fabulous!* (Philadelphia: Running Press, 2005).

Fruit and Vegetable Pesticide Load, www.sixwise.com/newsletters/07/06/13/the_20_fruits_and_vegetables_with_the_most_pesticides_the_20_with_the_least__and_what_to_do.htm.

Jamie Oliver Food Revolution, www.youtube.com/watch?v=S9B7im8aQjo.

La Maison Orphee Inc., First-cold-pressed oils, http://maisonorphee.com/en/.

Mayo Clinic, Basal Metabolic Rate, www.mayoclinic.com/health/metabolism/WT00006.

Pollan, Michael. *The Omnivore's Dilemma: A Natural History of Four Meals* (New York: Penguin, 2006).

Roizen, Michael F., MD and Mehmet C. Oz, MD, *YOU the Owner's Manual: An Insider's Guide to the Body That Will Make You Healthier and Younger* (New York: HarperResource, 2005).

Roizen, Michael F., MD, Mehmet C. Oz, MD, *YOU on a Diet: The Owner's Manual for Waist Management* (New York: Free Press, 2006).

Whole Grain Council, http://wholegrainscouncil.org/search/node/canada%20stamp.

Whole Grain Council, http://www.wholegrainscouncil.org/whole-grain-stamp/government-guidance.

About the Author

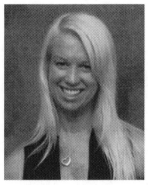 Nathalie loves people. She is genuinely interested in their behavior, understanding how they think, and listening to people's words, which represent their conception of their reality. She believes that the brain is the most complex structure in the universe and that we can all use it more, better, and differently. She knows that we all have everything we need, inside, to be our best. We can be who we choose to be—and that includes being healthy, happy, and feeling great!

She works as a Life Coach, one-on-one with clients, using Neuro-Linguistic-Programming (NLP) skills to help people find out what they want and achieve it. Whether it is losing the last ten pounds, finding a boyfriend, changing a bad habit, quitting smoking, fixing a relationship, advancing a career, getting pregnant, and so on, her clients are highly successful in achieving their goals.

Originally from Quebec City in Canada, she has been teaching fitness for twenty-four years. She lived in Toronto for eight years, where she taught for GoodLife Fitness and received the honor of being named Instructor of the Year for Canada in 2006 and was a Top 5 Instructor of the

Year finalist in 2008. Her husband and herself moved to British Columbia in 2009, where she still teaches fitness classes, as well as teaching Zumba locally in the White Rock community where they currently reside.

She has a Personal Training Specialist certification, which allows her to help her clients with personalized workout programs, and she is certified as a Nutrition and Wellness Specialist, which was mostly the basis for writing this book.

DON'T JUST BE. BE YOUR BEST!

Nathalie Plamondon-Thomas

Life Coach, Fitness Instructor Specialist, Personal Trainer,
Nutrition and Wellness Specialist, AIM, NLP, Zumba
Les Mills BODYATTACK, BODYPUMP, BODYFLOW,
BODYSTEP, BODYCOMBAT, BODYJAM, RPM
Newbody, Schwinn, Yoga, Resist-A-Ball, BOSU, Zumba, Gymstick,
Stott Pilates Foam Roller, Kettleball, Gliding, BodyFit
Top 5 Fitness Instructor of the Year 2008 for GoodLife Fitness Canada
Fitness Instructor of the Year 2006 for GoodLife Fitness Canada

DNA LIFE COACHING
Life Coaching, Personal Training, Fitness, Nutrition,
Weight Management, NLP, Zumba
www.dnalifecoaching.com
www.dnacoachdevie.com
nathalie@dnalifecoaching.com

THANKS TO . . .

Special thanks to Postcard Creative (www.postcardcreative.com) for assisting with the layout and editing of this book.

www.postcardcreative.com